# Other Books by the Author

Quick Headache Relief without Drugs
Back Pains, Quick Relief without Drugs

# Medical Dollar$ AND
# Life-Saving Sense

Howard D. Kurland, MD, DLFAPA

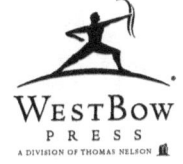

WESTBOW
PRESS
A DIVISION OF THOMAS NELSON

WestBow Press books may be ordered through booksellers or by contacting:

WestBow Press
A Division of Thomas Nelson
1663 Liberty Drive
Bloomington, IN 47403
www.westbowpress.com
1 (866) 928-1240

ISBN: 978-1-4908-1752-1 (sc)
ISBN: 978-1-4908-1753-8 (hc)
ISBN: 978-1-4908-1751-4 (e)

Library of Congress Control Number: 2013921124

Printed in the United States of America.

WestBow Press rev. date: 11/26/2013

And whoever saves a life, it is considered that he saved an entire world.

—Hillel, period of 30 BCE–10 CE

But how shall we expect charity towards others, when we are uncharitable to ourselves? Charity begins at home, is the voice of the world.

—Sir Thomas Browne, 1642

# Contents

1 Lifesaving........................................1

2 Sailing into Uncharted Waters..............5

3 Negotiating the Ladders: Basic Training....21

4 Anchors Aweigh: Sail On to Victory........27

5 Catching the Next Vessel....................35

6 Lost Horizons................................41

7 Shipwreck Benefits..........................49

8 Stormy Seas..................................55

9 Man Overboard!..............................61

10 Lost and Found.............................67

11    Shooting Star ⁓⁓⁓⁓⁓⁓⁓⁓⁓⁓⁓⁓ 71

12    Change of Course ⁓⁓⁓⁓⁓⁓⁓⁓⁓ 77

13    Vessel Sunk by Friendly Fire ⁓⁓⁓ 83

14    In Transit at an Idyllic Port ⁓⁓⁓⁓ 91

15    Twenty-One-Gun Salute ⁓⁓⁓⁓⁓ 97

16    Attention on Deck ⁓⁓⁓⁓⁓⁓⁓⁓ 103

17    Disembarkation ⁓⁓⁓⁓⁓⁓⁓⁓⁓ 107

18    Home Port ⁓⁓⁓⁓⁓⁓⁓⁓⁓⁓⁓ 113

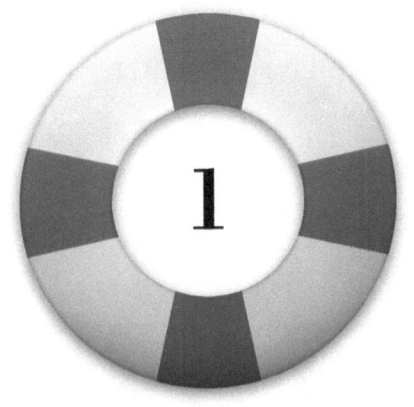

# 1     Lifesaving

In one format or another, the following parable merits frequent consideration.

A religious man stood on the roof of his house during a terrible flood. He prayed to the Lord for salvation. The waters were rising. Soon they would reach the roof of the house where he stood.

"Spare me, Lord," he pleaded fervently. "I have been a righteous man, and will continue to serve You well."

Soon a speedboat came by the roof. "Get in," shouted the captain of the speedboat.

But the righteous man responded loudly, "Save my neighbors on the roof of that house over there. The Lord will save me."

The waters were still slowly rising. Now the righteous man's feet were covered with a layer of water.

Shortly, another vessel approached. "Get aboard," the skipper commanded.

"No. Rescue that family over there," the righteous man responded. "The Lord will save me."

Now the floodwaters rose over the shoulders of the righteous man. As he struggled, he spotted yet another family on a distant rooftop. They were about to succumb to the flood. When the next rescue vessel arrived, the righteous man directed that vessel to save them. "The Lord will save me," he said.

Finally, the floodwaters engulfed the righteous man, and he was taken to his eternal reward.

The spirit of the righteous man was awarded an audience with the Lord. "I was righteous and faithful my entire life. How could You let me perish in the flood?"

The Lord responded, "Who let you drown? I sent three boats to rescue you!"

# Carry-Away Lifesavers

This book reveals real medical rescue vessels. You will be informed about essentials of basic examinations that should be requested but are frequently omitted. Modern translational medicine, which incorporates research into clinical practice, is presented. Combined neurobiological and psychological treatments are presented to illustrate effective medical therapeutics.

Specific, brief real-life accounts reveal how some utilize lifeboats and how others spurn rescue.

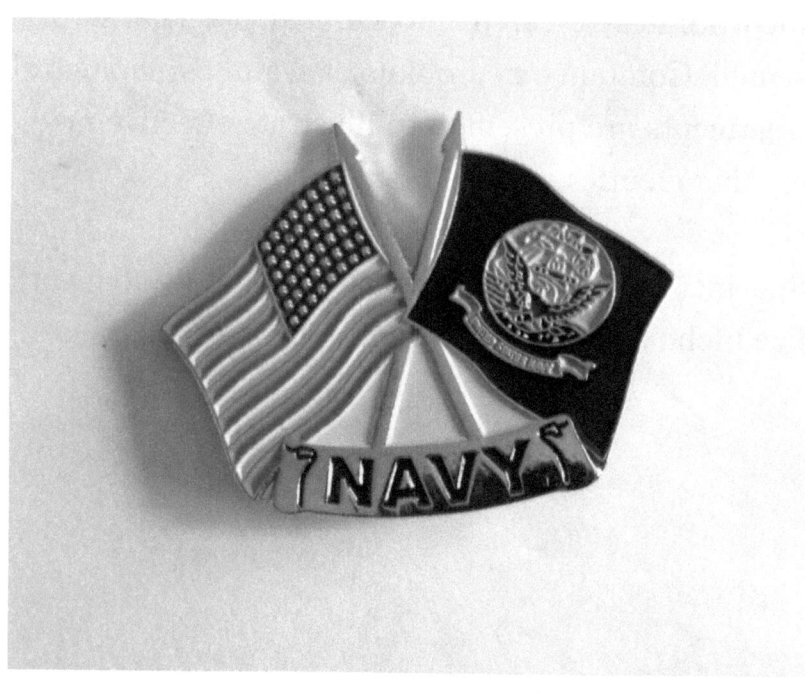

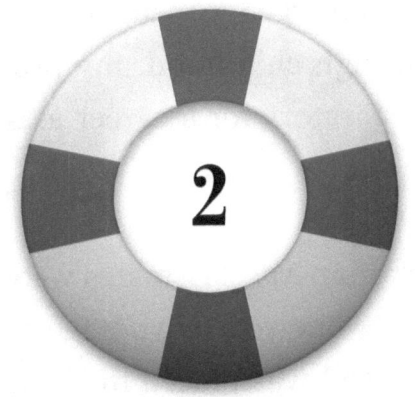

# Sailing into Uncharted Waters

**B**efore embarking on this voyage to elucidate medical issues pertinent to your health and welfare, you might wish to know a brief background of your cruise director.

My childhood was punctuated by multiple lifesaving rescues administered by a family doctor who made in-home visits (house calls) to administer treatment for acute asthmatic crises.

Refusing to be hostage to severe allergic asthma, I was very active in athletic activities with friends. Overexertion and outdoor allergies were effective triggers for asthmatic crises. I had to overcome my memories of frantic gasping for air many years later when I obtained certification for scuba diving.

Despite my gratitude for the emergency medical care that enabled me to get through childhood, my pre-college ambitions were preparatory for a career as a trial lawyer.

My parents were short in stature. My classmates were taller than I, and they had a one-year advantage in physical development because I was placed in grade school classes a full year ahead of my age peers. Therefore, I learned to defend myself both physically and verbally.

The husband of my mother's closest friend was an attorney. My theory was that he was grooming a prospective spouse for his daughter. At any rate, he inspired my involvement in debate. When he tragically perished suddenly at a young age, his will revealed that his entire law library was to be given to me when I started law school. We celebrated my acceptance to Dartmouth College, and I contemplated my prelaw studies.

The summer before my college admission, my mother contracted a serious ailment. It was not known how long it would take her to recover or if she could recover. Consequently, I exchanged my Ivy League education for a Midwestern education at Western Reserve (now Case-Reserve) University.

It was my good fortune and privilege to have the benefit of Calvin Hall, professor and head of the psychology department. Professor Hall allowed me take graduate courses in psychology as a junior college student. Instead of entering medical school after 3 rather than the usual 4 years of college (a procedure termed "in absentia"} an agreement was made with Northwestern University Medical School that I would matriculate there after completion of my fourth year of college.

My senior year of college, I completed my graduate studies in psychology. I was elected to Psi Chi, the graduate scholastic honorary society. Professor Hall did not advise my staying an additional year to complete the doctoral thesis necessary to obtain a PhD in psychology. His counsel that an MD degree would suffice proved correct.

My clinical medical education was superb. My efforts were rewarded with election to AOA, the medical scholastic honorary. In the year of my graduation, the most highly regarded residencies in the specialty of internal medicine appeared to be in New York, at Mt. Sinai Medical Center. I was assigned to a general rotating medical internship at Mt. Sinai Hospital in Cleveland preparatory to residency training in New York.

Having been raised in Shaker Heights, a suburb of Cleveland, I hoped to return to my hometown to establish a private practice of internal medicine. An internship in Cleveland would allow me to establish connections to expedite setting up a practice there after a residency on the East Coast.

During my internship in Cleveland, another life-changing event occurred. My mother had re-covered from her previous illness. Driving in her automobile, a drunk driver demolished her vehicle. She was sent to the ER of the hospital where I was interning. Several days later, my mother was still hospitalized there as an inpatient.

I was resting in my room, while the medical staff attended to her. When there was no EKG or EEG evidence of life, she was pronounced dead. I was told that, if I requested it, they would permit her to remain in her room so that I could view her before she was removed to the morgue.

In a very unprofessional manner, I ran to my mother's hospital room. In a frenzied state, I shouted an order to a floor nurse to prepare an injection of Aramine, a heart stimulant. The nurse complied, most probably out of respect for a crazed intern who had just lost his mother.

I plunged the needle through the chest wall into my mother's heart muscle. There was no response. I repeated the procedure with a second and then a third injection through the chest wall.

Following the third injection, the nurse tearfully stated she could no longer cooperate. But moments later, the unimaginable occurred: my mother awakened. She related that she had witnessed the entire medical episode as she floated in a white cloud near the ceiling of the room. She recalled the flatline EKG and the death pronouncement.

The respected chairman of medicine had witnessed the flat EKGs for thirty minutes and pronounced the death. My mother witnessed the discussion about notifying me before removing her body to the morgue. She observed the Aramine injections that I administered through her chest wall. The episode was vividly recalled by my mother until her final demise some twenty-five years later.

That episode was life-changing for both my mother and myself. After serious contemplation of the meaning of such a momentous occasion, I concurred with the advice of my medical mentors. Although it was agreed that I could be a competent internal medical specialist, the unanimous opinion was that my contribution to neuropsychiatry would probably be far more valuable. I had a background in psychology and had initiated inquiry into the neuroendocrinology of depression while in medical school. The neuropsychiatry residency affiliated with my medical school promptly accepted me for the first year of training.

During my first year of residency, I was able to convince the US Naval Reserve to accept me (despite my asthma history and 4-F draft classification) as a reserve medical officer. Once I had obtained reserve medical officer status and had served for several months, I applied to finish my last two years of neuropsychiatric residency in the navy.

I was privileged to receive orders to the Naval Medical Hospital in Oakland, California. At that medical facility, there was a medical research facility named the Clinical Investigation Center. At that time, the director was CDR. Raymond Watten. The chairman of the research advisory committee was the dean of UC San Francisco Medical School, Professor Harold Harper. These gentlemen approved funding and space for a lowly second-year resident.

Shortly after starting my training in the navy, there was a scientific article published that outlined a laboratory technique enabling the practical identification of urinary corticosteroids.

I prepared a research protocol to measure urinary corticosteroid output. Comparison of corticosteroid output from depressed patients with that from healthy controls could elucidate the involvement of adrenal corticosteroid function in depression. While in medical school, I had discussed this hypothesis with leading endocrinologists. They had dismissed it as nonsense, and I had been unable to pursue the research.

When carefully controlled studies in my navy CIC lab revealed abnormalities of adrenal hyperfunction in depressed patients, I published several papers on it in medical journals. The navy sent me to lecture at Walter Reed Army Hospital in Washington, DC, and at the National Institutes of Health in Bethesda. My research was replicated by the then-director of NIMH. Thereafter, NIMH began to study depression in addition to their previous principal focus on schizophrenia.

Success with steroid research enabled expansion into multiple other aspects of neuropsychiatry. One of those was in the utilization of the newly developed computer analysis of EEGs. With the collaboration and tutelage of Professor Charles Yeager, I researched the effects of psychedelic drugs on computer-analyzed electric brain activity and published my findings in the scientific literature. After I presented that material to the Pan-American Medical Association, I was made a Life Fellow of the PAMA.

While on active duty in the navy, my neck and lower back were injured severely while traveling on orders. I recovered from the acute disability but was left with lifetime limitations. I had been promoted from reserve to regular navy, and my rank was promoted to lieutenant commander. My next duty station was to take command of a neuropsychiatric facility in Japan, with the prospect of promotion to commander.

However, my spine was no longer well-suited for overseas duty. An unsolicited offer had been made by my medical school, Northwestern, to accept the position of head of neurology and psychiatry at the VA Research Hospital, which then served as the university teaching hospital. (Passavant and Wesley Hospitals were on campus, but they were considered private hospitals that hosted NU residents.)

The opportunity to chair a department at a university hospital and be a voting member on the dean's committee would ordinarily require twenty years more medical experience than I had. It therefore became an irresistible opportunity. I would not leave government service; I would just transfer from USN to VA. But I would be a head of neurology and psychiatry in a university hospital and a member of the dean's committee.

After four plus years of active duty, I was discharged from the navy with a partial disability because of my back injuries.

When I commenced the position as chief of a university hospital neuropsychiatric residency program, I was amazed to discover that a formal didactic curriculum was not in place. The teaching program was limited to clinical rotations, supervision, and, in some cases, conferences.

With all possible deliberation and speed, I established a comprehensive didactic curriculum, recruited specialized practitioners from the Chicago area, and commenced a comprehensive residency training program.

The response was overwhelming in the recruitment of new, high-quality residents. We had to obtain additional funding to handle the enlarged residency loads. Other hospitals in the immediate area were not able to fill their minimum resident quotas, and they attempted to bargain for our seeming oversupply.

My four-year tenure running that hospital service was concurrent with being a full-time medical school assistant and then associate professor. But several new factors arose. There was a position of associate dean of the medical school that was becoming vacant, and I was asked to apply for it.

I was complimented that the opportunity was made available, but I was not desirous of a life in management rather than medicine. While I had no problem with research funding in the navy, VA central officials made a site visit to confront me.

Those central office representatives informed me that they would deny funding for my current research. They stated that the studies were unrealistic and could not be done. When I displayed published papers in peer-reviewed medical journals, they were dismissed with disbelief. According to unofficial comments from other officials, my reviewers were several decades older than I and were incensed that the VA was compensating me in a higher pay grade. I later learned that an official publication had revealed that an employee of less than thirty years of age was receiving top-grades compensation.

And so it was time to set sail from full-time academia to full-time private practice and part-time professorship. Moreover, my physical status had changed significantly. My back problems became progressively more troublesome. I developed severe sciatic pain and back spasm, but I would not take pain medications or spasm-relief agents, because I wanted to practice medicine with an un-drugged sensorium. My orthopedic surgeon informed me that my problems were too extensive.

At that point in time, there were no appropriate surgical remedies available. Consequently, I was fitted with back braces. The final version was a metal back brace. The frame of the metal brace was held by heavy elastic and straps that secured the brace over my back and by bindings over my abdominal wall up to my chest cavity. I had been consigned to a life in a medieval torture device. I walked stiffly with the aid of a cane.

Meanwhile, Ray Watten had been promoted to captain and sent to command the research facility in Taipei, Taiwan. He wrote to me about a Chinese employee who had attempted to utilize a treatment little known to Westerners at the time.

The treatment had enabled the employee to get off the narcotics which had been previously required to alleviate severe arthritic pains. The new treatment was called acupuncture. There was hope for me.

My first exposure to acupuncture treatment took place in a fly-infested second-floor clinic over a grocery store. The sterilized needles that we brought were inserted by unsterile, unclean fingers.

Nevertheless, I walked up the stairs to that clinic wearing my metal back brace. I walked down the stairs after the initial treatment holding the brace in my hands.

More important than just relieving my own pain, I now had a mission to acquire new skills to relieve the pain of others. I traveled throughout Japan, China, Thailand, and the Philippines to learn more.

Thereafter, I attempted to integrate oriental medicine with Western medical neurology. I observed many practitioners who performed acupuncture stimulation with finger pressure. But I never observed anyone teaching the patient how to use pressure points on themselves, nor was I able to find anything in print at that time that promoted self-treatment.

Therefore, I devised a self-treatment technique for headache relief. I tested the technique on headache patients and found it effective. The book entitled Quick Headache Relief without Drugs was published in many languages. When an editor of

Book-of-the-Month followed the instructions and got migraine relief, it became an alternate selection of Book-of-the-Month Club. The National Hospital for Neurology and Neurosurgery in Queen's Square, London, for many years distributed (with my permission) copies of chapters from the book to patients.

Although the concept of auto-acupressure is my invention and my copyright, you may now find literally hundreds of books espousing self-administered acupressure techniques. Wonderful. The word got around.

As stated above, I gave my permission for medical centers to distribute the technique without charge. Throughout the orient, the concept of auto-acupressure was very well accepted. I was invited to lecture in numerous locations and was the principal speaker at the East-West Pain Conference, Xian, China. My work with graduate students in the department of physiology of the University of Hong Kong was especially rewarding.

Sometimes, my visiting-professor lectures resulted in unexpectedly valuable outcomes. A fellow psychiatrist, Dr. Donja Barr, heard me lecture at the Cook

County School of Medicine. She referred her husband, Bill Barr, for treatment of phantom limb pain secondary to traumatic amputation of a leg. Acupuncture treatments could relieve his stump pain only temporarily because (we discovered) his prosthesis was faulty. Also, the surgical amputation repair proved faulty. (Bill Barr's book Whole Again describes many of the events related to his traumatic amputation and subsequent struggles to recover his life.)

One evening a problem-solving dinner was held, and the result was the establishment of the Institute for Advancement of Prosthetics. The institute employed the most outstanding prosthetist—Jan Stakosa. CAD-CAM (computer-aided design and computer-aided manufacturing) of prosthetics was pushed into the mainstream. The Ertl procedure for limb amputations was made available to major trauma centers around the world both by live demonstration and videotape.

The institute addressed the lack of training and standards for prosthetists by having Medicare and Medicaid establish requirements for reimbursement. On a state level, an attempt was made to have each state adopt licensure standards.

My book publishers enticed me into doing national tours to appear on local and national radio and television by accepting the condition that I traveled with my wife. School obligations often prevented our children from joining us.

Publishers requested the promotion of my new hardcover book and then again when the paperback edition appeared; however, parental responsibilities made my withdrawal from broadcast/world touring circuits necessary. Enjoying the presence of children and grandchildren is the richest of life's experiences.

It is time for us to leave these glimpses into my background and embark on your educational cruise.

# Negotiating the Ladders: Basic Training

## 3

On a naval vessel there are no stairways. One descends to the lower deck or ascends to the upper deck by traversing ladders. The act of climbing up or climbing down the ladders is described as "negotiating the ladders." Failure to learn how to quickly and safely negotiate ladders may cause the loss of life and limb. Failure to secure a hatch promptly could cause the loss of the vessel.

When you are "aboard" a medical visit, you are responsible to negotiate quickly. Your concerns must be made known in a timely fashion. Many patients are embarrassed to initially discuss their most vital concerns, usually waiting until the end of an appointment before inquiring about that "one more thing." In this current world of managed care (and especially

"Obamacare"), the time may not be available to discuss that "one last thing."

There are essentials of health that should always be evaluated. The body (and brain) do not function without adequate blood supply. If your blood pressure is too high or too low, there are problems. If your blood pressure is acceptable when you are seated, it should also be acceptable when you are standing.

Emotional stressors may drastically elevate standing blood pressures. Lack of sleep quantity and quality may decrease initial standing blood pressures. Low sodium levels may cause dangerously low standing pressures, and these often accentuate the drop in pressure on arising.

Orthostatic hypotension (abnormally low pressure on standing up) is frequently related to carotid sinus sensitivity (diminished response of the pressure sensors in the main neck arteries) in all age groups. Orthostatic hypotension is a cardinal symptom of neurodegenerative diseases, such as Parkinson's syndrome.

Do not leave the doctor's office without assessment of heart rate, heart rhythm, and blood pressure.

Do not fall prey to the assumption that no blood tests are required because you are not aware of signs or symptoms. For example, low vitamin D levels are associated with increased risk of developing multiple sclerosis as well as with exacerbating the severity of the illness. Current research has shown suboptimal performance of the brain, bone, and heart with vitamin D deficiency.

Most of my patients do not have vitamin D levels requested by their internists. The hospital lab informed me that Medicare and most insurance companies will not cover the cost of the test unless the physician has specifically coded the lab requisition with a deficiency diagnostic code.

In my well-fed patient population, almost all the adults who did not take supplements and did not subsist on milk products had abnormally low vitamin D levels.

Highly significant information is readily available just by observation of the manner of rising up from the seated position and walking. Was this done?

Frequently, balance problems become evident when a person is challenged to stand on one foot, and these may become more prominent when eyes are closed.

When vitamin B12 levels are deficient and there is an impairment of sensation input in the nerves from the foot, a condition called neurologic PA (pernicious anemia) may be suspect. In such cases, significant neurological damage occurs before anemia becomes clinically apparent. This occurs frequently enough to be included on the list of essential examinations.

If a problem with an endocrine gland, such as the thyroid, is diagnosed, inquire whether the tests ordered are sufficiently comprehensive.

For example, the TSH (thyroid-stimulating hormone) and T4 levels may be normal, but the T3 level may be low and indicative of T3 hypothyroidism. Weight gain, leg edema, and emotional depression may be symptoms of T3 hypothyroidism that has gone undiagnosed because of normal TSH and T4 levels.

Recently, the substitution of generic thyroid medications has produced a significant number of patients with T3 hypothyroidism.

Observation of your demeanor, skin tone, and general appearance may be diagnostic, especially if your physician is rendering ongoing care. In an initial encounter, a physician may not appreciate that your usual jovial mood is absent, that you appear paler than usual, and that your unique manner of dress is absent.

When your consultation is an annual checkup for physical status, examination with a light in eyes, ear canals, and the oral cavity, is essential. Melanomas and other skin tumors can occur on any part of the anatomy, and detection of these requires a full-body inspection. Other body cavities also require appropriate examination that otherwise would be considered an invasion of privacy.

Accuracy and completeness stack the deck in your favor. If you fail to reveal illness symptoms and family medical problems, your opportunity for diagnosis and treatment may be compromised.

Allow the physician to develop a medical diagnosis independently. If you overemphasize a main complaint, it may distract the diagnosis of a related condition, causal factors, or other medical problems. The main complaint is not always the most significant.

The nature of the problem should dictate the frequency of appointments. If you are afflicted with a serious depression and require the initiation of medication, your follow-up should be measured in days rather than weeks or months. If you have severe hypertension requiring the initiation of a medicine titration, there is a significant risk of damage if the follow-up is delayed for a quarter of a year.

You have successfully negotiated the ladders to the sunny decks when your medical consultation provides you with the comfort that your complaints are being reasonably evaluated and treatment options delineated.

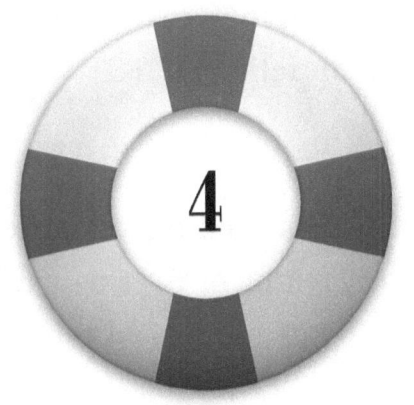

# 4

# Anchors Aweigh:
# Sail On to Victory

A seventy-six-year-old widowed mother of seven children was happily remarried. She had recently had a surgical procedure to correct a painful knee condition. The surgery involved a general anesthesia without complications.

Shortly following the surgery, it was noticeable that the patient failed to recover her energy, vigor, motivation, appetite, and enthusiasm for life. She began to demonstrate hand trembling and walked with a rigid, stiff posture.

A neurologist was consulted who diagnosed Parkinson's disease, and the woman started an antitremor medication (Sinemet; generic: carbidopa-levodopa). High blood pressure was also diagnosed, for which an antihypertensive heart medication (lisinopril) and diuretic (HCTZ) were prescribed.

Moreover, the presence of clinical neuropsychiatric depression was recognized. Treatment for this was initiated with a modern antidepressant medication (venlafaxine).

Despite having clinical depression, hypertension, and Parkinson's disease all correctly diagnosed, and despite the initiation of appropriate pharmacological treatment, the patient continued to have unrelenting depression, unrelieved tremors and stiffness, and progressive impairment in memory recall over the next two months.

This deterioration especially alarmed one of her step-daughters, who brought her concerns about her new mother to me and requested my opinions. It was the urging of the stepdaughter that motivated the con-sultation with me.

At our first meeting her primary concern was "de-pression"; however, in the following two months she continued to have such poor appetite that she had lost twenty-six pounds. My patient did not complain of sleep difficulties, but she was beset with feelings of nervousness, depression, difficulty in decision making, increased irritability, incessant worrying, and constant fatigue.

Repeated questions after hearing both short and lengthy replies to her inquiries revealed rather profound short-term memory impairment.

When I observed her movement, it revealed a marked rigidity and shuffling gait. There were intermittent tremors at rest of the fingers and limbs. Her handwriting revealed the micographia (small letters) commonly found in Parkinson patients. There were significant difficulties in maintaining balance while walking, but these were especially noticeable when she attempted to maintain balance with her eyes closed. There was some minor intention tremor noted on the finger-to-nose pointing test. Generally, her motor defects revealed a small amount of cerebellar dysfunction but a large amount of basal ganglia-related Parkinson's disorder.

I also discovered a significantly elevated systolic hypertension. Sitting systolic blood pressures were in the 170 range. Persistent, nonexercise blood pressures over

140 are associated with brain white matter (and sometimes gray matter) damage. Such damage may lead to progressive mental decline (dementia) as well as stroke.

My recommendations for treatment modifications followed an explanation of the larger picture of developing illnesses. Most probably aggravated by high blood pressure, the response to a surgical procedure and general anesthesia was an acceleration of cerebral neurodegeneration.

Parkinson's disease is a neurodegenerative disorder of the basal ganglia in the brain stem, with a loss of dopamine in the substantia nigra nuclei. However, the most destructive factor for many lives is not the tremor disorder but the cognitive disorder and resultant dementia.

Neurophysiological healing requires restoration of normal brain chemistry. The absence of adequate amounts of vitamin B12 and methylfolate (the brain-active form of the folic acid B vitamin) can result in enormous dysfunction.

Low B12 levels often are associated with cerebellar problems. In severe neurological pernicious anemia, there is significant impairment of memory. Antidepressant medication and antitremor medications often work more swiftly and effectively when they are augmented with methylfolate.

Newer medications that are derived for active isomers and/or active metabolic derivatives of approved medications may be more effective and may have fewer undesirable side effects.

Previously, the antidepressant venlafaxine was employed in a starting dosage. In my opinion, its newer derivative desvenlafaxine (Pristiq) is a superior agent.

Consequently, the first changes in medication that I recommended were the addition of daily doses 1000 mcg of B12, 15 mg of methylfolate, and the substitution of 50 mg of desvenlefaxine for the venlefaxine. I also reminded the patient to involve internal medicine, emphasizing the need for cardiologists to monitor the antihypertensive medications.

Because of the patient's planned return to an out-of-state residence, she scheduled the follow-up appointment just six days later. It was difficult to believe what I observed and heard. There was significant subjective and objective improvement. Depression was mostly lifted, and hand tremors were about 80 percent decreased. It was amazing!

As expected, the short-term memory impairment was still significant. The systolic hypertension remained. I gave instructions to begin a titration dosage of a memory-enhancing, neuroprotective medication named memantadine (Namenda). Usage of this medication has multiple decades of proven clinical effectiveness in my practice. Frequently it is necessary to add other memory-neuroprotective agents such as donepezil (Aricept). But adding Namenda after Aricept often produces little discernible clinical improvement, unlike the reverse order.

After completing the initial dosing of Namenda, during the following months, the larger maintenance dose was prescribed for morning and evening. Antihypertensive medications were adjusted. Life went on as before.

Five months later, her stepdaughter told me that her mother wasn't going to follow-up appointments because her mother said, "There is nothing wrong. I'm my old self."

Our discussions helped the mother realize that the stepdaughter was a valuable family member, so she had become a "daughter." Perhaps life turned out better than expected.

## Carry-Away Lifesavers

Every time a person has surgery with anesthesia, the body organ called the brain is affected. The amount of the effect depends upon the nature of the surgery, the nature of the anesthesia, and the preexisting physical and psychological conditions of the patient.

Recovery times from serious ailments are usually measured with a calendar, not a stopwatch. But if your progress is stalled and recovery is not progressing as expected, reevaluation is appropriate.

Hold true to course. If yet another treatment will make things even better, take the blessed thing.

The determining test is the ability to hold to the course once it feels like full recovery has put the wind back in your sails.

# 5

# Catching the Next Vessel

Sometimes the vehicle that speeds recovery comes out of the fog.

A psychotherapist became overwhelmed by his own problems in the course of advancing age and declining health. His introduction into the golden Medicare years was painful. He suffered a heart attack (myocardial infarction). He had an angioplasty, and doctors inserted drug-eluting stents in his coronary arteries.

Psychiatric depression consumed his every waking moment. His self-consumption was almost total. His suffering was painful to observers. No day was completed without a multiplicity of panic attacks and "adrenaline surges" that punctuated the underlying and ever-present depression.

As if the emotional distress was not sufficient, there was constant fearfulness about a recent heart attack that had necessitated the placement of stents in his coronary arteries. His sleep was interrupted with frequent awakening accompanied by terrible nightmares and sensations of painful experiences that felt like ice water and electricity.

Antianxiety and antidepressant medications were initiated. Unfortunately, whatever was prescribed did not immediately relieve all the agonizing symptoms. One medication after another was blamed for the same symptoms for which it had been prescribed. Necessary titrations (increases of dosage) were rejected.

Although small doses of medication did provide some symptomatic improvement, residual symptomatology was ascribed to the meds. It was not possible to obtain adequate progress without meaningful levels of medication, and terrible suffering persisted. Psychological therapy was held hostage by physiological imbalance.

Fearing catastrophic emotional and physical consequences, I discussed the use of alternative proven treatments for severe depression. We discussed studies that documented decreased life spans of eight to nine years in patients with untreated bipolar disorder.

ECT (electroconvulsive treatment) has had decades of proven effectiveness. It remains a current recommendation of US and international medical societies.

Back in 1959, impressed by the work of a pioneering anesthesiologist (Dr. Herbert Epstein) and psychiatrist (Dr. Meyer Brown), I compiled the data on their first five thousand treatments. ECT was given with anesthesia without significant morbidity (ill effect) in five thousand treatments. We published that study, which was the first of its kind.

More than fifty years later, ECT with anesthesia remains a medical staple. Back in the days of Hippocrates, electric eels probably set the stage for the development of ECT.

In modern times, two Italian physicians, Cerletti and Bini, are generally credited for the early development of ECT. Convulsions were often observed to cause the remission of depressive symptoms in diabetics who experienced seizures from low blood sugar (hypoglycemia). Before the development of ECT, insulin convulsive therapy was utilized, but ECT was much safer and easier to administer.

As circumstance would have it, there was no inpatient bed space available to my patient to begin ECT. Several weeks passed, and the fear of the ECT grew as great as the fear of medications. In the weeks of waiting, medical evaluation continued—and a new vessel appeared.

A tangle of rapidly-growing blood vessels appeared on the undersurface of the third rib: a type of tumor known as a hemangioma. The patient swiftly agreed to surgery.

General anesthesia was required for a thoracotomy (chest wall surgery). The surgeon opened the anterior chest wall, removed the blood vessel tumor, and then reconstructed the chest wall.

Following that major surgery, the patient accepted pain medication, along with some minor tranquilizers and small doses of an antidepressant. Psychotherapy for depression resumed.

Less than half of the psychiatric symptoms of depression remained, and those symptoms were much more tolerable after surviving the surgical removal of the (benign) chest wall blood vessel tumor. Without the arrival of those vessels, the desire to recover from depression would not have appeared.

## Carry-Away Lifesavers

With persistence, the proper vehicle for your recovery may be found.

The vessel that provides your recovery may not be the one that you expected. You must utilize that vessel so you can sight the next horizon.

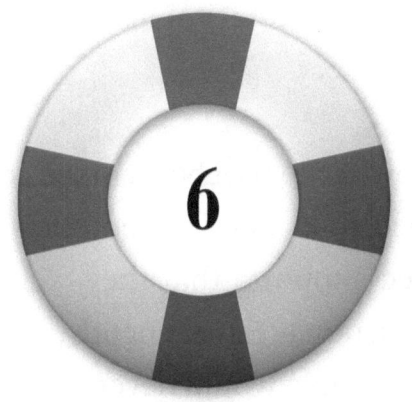

# 6     Lost Horizons

This patient came from a very modest northeast community and had a master's degree in bio-chemistry, but she had recently been doing doctor-ate-level research for a prestigious national firm. She had married a physician who also shared her research interests. They had recently moved from the East because her husband accepted a prestigious position at a major Chicago medical center.

Despite all these achievements, she was hostage to abdominal infirmities, and she was a frequent visitor to the offices of gastroenterologists.

During their previous residency in New York, they had received marital counseling which addressed her desire to conceive. The husband was only interested in one child, and he had this child from his first marriage. He had revoked his premarital agreement to have kids with his new wife.

It is difficult to imagine how some psychotherapeutic direction was not provided to resolve the conflicts, but the historical evidence supports that they were not provided necessary assistance. Subsequently, the seemingly happily married couple would never attain the richness and fulfillment of a family life that they both desired.

They both continued to enjoy professional success. Her achievements as a research biochemist were supported by evening tutorials from the physician husband. But her motherly desires went unfulfilled. Occasional visits from the stepson provided scant fulfillment. She was not the biological mother and was regarded only as a new companion of the father.

The consequence was symptoms of psychiatric depression. Cloudy moods cast their shadows over most days despite the radiance of marriage and professional success.

She developed a friendship with a research assistant colleague at work after a lunch cafeteria discussion.

Both her new friend and her brother had survived the Holocaust in Europe as rescued children from camps where the parents perished. The woman's new girlfriend was enjoying her adult years after much psychotherapeutic endeavor. Eagerly relating her success in overcoming Holocaust-related trauma, she urged her new biochemist friend to seek consultation in my office.

A very proper and stylish lady scientist appeared in my office, displaying the quiet dignity of a successful corporate image. But her medical and psychiatric difficulties were substantial. My first task was to assure her that she would be treated as physically ill, not psychoneurotic, during the new medical referrals that we would arrange.

As is commonly seen, the combination of appropriate psychiatric medication and psychological problem-solving enabled a change in perspective. The couple's marital communication improved, and affection returned. She began to enjoy life, and her resentments were put into perspective.

Several decades passed with ever-increasing enjoyment of her marriage. Ongoing efforts with the stepson brought some improvement, but never a mother-child relationship.

During the next twenty years, their marriage continued to grow as a harmonious interdependence. Then catastrophe struck. After an acute coronary occlusion (heart attack), her spouse spent his dying days in a hospital bed bemoaning his failure to keep his vow to have children in his second marriage.

The attempt to unburden his guilt on his deathbed left the grieving spouse with memories of many happy years marred by a gaping wound of unfilled dreams. Life was better together than it would have been apart, but the empty void of the family that would never be forever lurked in the background of the sunniest of days.

The life of this widow was forever changed. She was already past retirement age but maintained many friendships from past work years. However, her empty apartment at night made her feel the absence of immediate family.

She placed an emergency call to my office one evening. I recall being alarmed when she related symptoms of confusion, unstable gait, and visual blurring. My long acquaintance with her medical care convinced me that her problem was neurological rather than psychological and that they required immediate attention in an emergency room.

Prompt medical evaluation in the ER and radiology departments revealed the cause of the symptoms. There was increased intracranial pressure secondary to an internal hydrocephalus. Emergency neurosurgery was performed, with placement of a stent to alleviate the increased intracranial fluid accumulation.

After post-surgical rehabilitation, she returned home to reside alone. Her mental function remained exceptional. Her strength resumed, and physical activities returned to previous levels.

She decided to remedy her lonely life with a move to a retirement facility, and she selected a location near a suburban city center. Now the library and the grocery were within walking distance. In addition, she would no longer be so isolated and would be able to give up her automobile.

This woman spent several pleasant years in the retirement home. She made new friends and enjoyed activities and the opportunity for communal dining. There were rentable rooms in the retirement facility to accommodate visitation for out-of-town friends, and in-town friends could be accommodated in the facility dining room. Life was better with others.

During the seventy-ninth and eightieth years of her life, she was besieged by multiple physical ailments. Her intestines became intolerant of her usual diet. Until we got her to the proper specialist, she spent months when proximity to a toilet was an activity determinant. She had an additional source of abdominal discomfort that was discovered to be related to a "female" problem. That was resolved with another surgery.

However, the physical pains and restriction of activities was fertile ground to regrow the memories of the lost opportunities for having a family. She was consumed with an overwhelming anger about her trusted spouse revoking his pledge to parent her kids. For many months, she ruminated constantly about her lost opportunities, repeatedly debating whether she should have left him in the early years to seek another mate. Once again, the dark clouds of depression engulfed her.

With psychotherapy sessions twice weekly for several months and the regulation of some neurochemical agents, she achieved reasonable perspective and resumed more normal social activities.

All the stressors took their toll. Signs of neurodegenerative disease interfered with some recent memory and decreased physical vigor. Her systolic blood pressure began to be episodically elevated to dangerous levels. At visits to her internist, the blood pressure elevations were minimized because of her advanced age.

A massive stroke sent her to her eternal reward during her eightieth year of life.

## Carry-Away Lifesavers

Make every reasonable effort to achieve life goals.

Actively confront obstacles in a timely fashion.

Surrendering the opportunity to bear children may produce irreconcilable regret.

If you seek professional guidance and feel you have failed to obtain it, attempt to find better qualified sources.

Regaining realistic perspective often permits visualizing the rainbow after the most terrible storms.

7        **Shipwreck Benefits**

A married woman in her midfifties was overcome by negativity and depression. She related an inability to cope with upcoming surgery to remove a large, cancerous tumor in her abdomen. She requested help to deal with overwhelming fears.

Although she was taking potent antihypertensive and diuretic medication (amlodipine and spironolactone), her systolic blood pressures were elevated to the 170 range. The effect of her anxieties on heart and blood vessels presented another significant medical danger.

We prepared her psychologically for the surgery, which was to be an abdominal procedure. That surgery was compared to the experience of giving birth to her 2 children. After completion of the surgery, she would then be able to enjoy forthcoming marriage of one child and the birth of a grandchild from another.

We reduced her anxieties and depression with the prescription of a tranquilizing antidepressant (trazodone).

Six weeks later, a despondent survivor of seven hours of abdominal surgery tearfully related that the tumor could not be entirely removed surgically. A malignant sarcoma was wrapped around major blood vessels and had infiltrated the retroperitoneal areas. She had been informed of a very dire, short-term prognosis. Her doctors said the tumor was untreatable and incurable.

She started taking a new antidepressant medication, Lexapro (escitalopram). We continued to increase the dosage of Lexapro to more therapeutic levels and continued with weekly psychotherapy. Her perspective improved, her mood brightened, and her anxieties diminished.

However, within the next month, the abdominal pains became so severe that she spent her daytimes at home, paralyzed with the dread of her impending painful demise.

Listening to the nature of the pain complaint, my presumptive diagnosis was that the severe abdominal pain was radiating from the back and coming from the spinal nerves. We discussed the use of laser bio-stimulation (laser acupuncture) as an immediately available, noninvasive technique for diagnosis and treatment.

Spinal nerve root involvement was identified with laser biostimulation, and it was traced around to the site of excruciating abdominal pains.

Selected laser frequencies associated with the relief of pain were applied, reducing inflammation and re-laxing the muscles of her affected areas. That single session provided significant physical pain relief and also provided even greater psychological relief from related fears. It also helped to rekindle the willing-ness to reconsider better times.

Prior to the discovery of her fatal illness, her life had been clouded over by her mother's unrelenting memories of surviving the Holocaust in Europe. Overwhelming pessimism drained the pleasures of her precancer existence. Only because of her deadly tumor did she accept referral for psychiatric treatment. During the post-cancer diagnosis and treatment years, she was able to experience some of the happiest years of her lifetime.

Previously embittered and scornful of religion, her perspective on life and the possibility of an afterlife were reshaped. After our discussions of such events as the one witnessed and described in chapter 2, religious support became an available asset. She sought additional pastoral counseling and engaged in further religious education. Her improved mood and perspective allowed her to have the best-ever relationship with her mother, enjoy her marital roles, and improve her relationship with her children.

Her prognosis for cancer survival had initially been about six months. Nevertheless, she experienced the happiest years of her life before the malignant sarcoma took her life about five years later.

# Carry-Away Lifesavers

Even the most calamitous adversity may propel you to happier destinations.

Keeping watch on the heavens has guided many ships to sunnier turf.

Especially in the prospect of impending shipwreck, the salvage value merits consideration. It may be the most valuable cargo of the voyage.

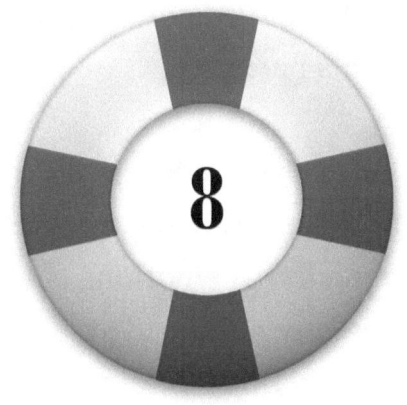

# 8     Stormy Seas

A young woman presented as a referral from a distinguished psychologist-psychotherapist. Despite his considerable skills, he was certain that this patient would not recover without neuropsychiatric medication.

Her anxieties were overwhelming. She had been the victim of severe marital abuse—both psychological and physical. Following one of the many times her husband expounded on the details of the latest plan to murder her, she realized that she had to escape. The agony was having to leave two young children without their biological mother.

She did escape. Her husband remarried. To the best of my knowledge, there are now four abused ex-wives.

Reconnection with her kids came in later decades, but that is getting ahead of this narrative.

Emotional pain, depression, and anxiety related to the situation were drowning the grieving mother. The physiological response to all this emotional suffering was evident with the greatly increased systolic blood pressures. Readings over 300 were present (rather than the expected 120s range). The physical danger of this much hypertension necessitated hospitalization.

There was excessive emotional distress that precluded placement on a medical unit, so she was admitted as an inpatient not to my neurology service, but to my psychiatry service.

My operative suspicion was that the extreme agitation so overwhelmed the adrenal gland that there was an excess secretion of hormone. If that was true, there might be a tumor called a pheochromocytoma. I ordered appropriate urine and blood tests and requested the consultation of an endocrinologist.

The endocrinologist did not think I was correct, and he canceled a CT that I had requested to attempt visualization of a possible pheochromocytoma. He persisted in this imperious behavior and canceled the CT a second time after I reordered it. With the consent of the suffering patient, the CT was once again reordered.

The CT demonstrated the presence of the adrenal tumor. Subsequent surgical removal revealed the presence of a large pheochromocytoma. Reevaluation of the urine studies revealed an error in the laboratory process, which had obscured the clinical diagnosis.

The patient's life had been saved, but her emotional distress had not been cured. However, after surgery, she was physically able to confront her emotional issues.

If the loss of a marriage and the parenting of two young children was not trauma enough, her family of origin provided even more grief. Without the complications of detail, it is accurate to state that fatal tragedies took her parents and alienated her brother.

Almost three decades later, a happily remarried, successful businesswoman enjoys parent and grandparent contact related to that first marriage. She still benefits from quarterly visits to regain perspective and to establish new strategies for confrontation of current issues.

Interestingly, her emotional stability and current blood pressure issues still require the use of anticonvulsant medication. That medication is Neurontin (gabapentin). With dosing throughout each day, both her anxieties and her blood pressure are controlled. Without it, neither is controlled.

The generic version of this medicine (gabapentin) did not that have that effect. Apparently she was allergic to a substance in the binder of the generic. The name brand medication (Neurontin) continues its decades of efficacy. The generic was toxic.

# Carry-Away Lifesavers

The will to survive may overcome the stormiest of seas.

The will to thrive may overcome the worst shipwrecks.

Happiness can come to those who work to achieve it.

Emotional illness does not mean there are no bodily disorders.

Overcoming emotional illness often requires treating both body and brain.

If a medication is the correct one for you, use it. Do not abandon a medication because the generic substitution is not acceptable.

# 9    Man Overboard!

In the midst of an income tax–preparation season, a successful CPA was referred by his internal medical doctor to assist in obtaining relief from unbearable back pain.

MRI imaging had revealed significant spinal disease throughout the lumbar spine and especially from the fourth lumbar to the first sacral vertebrae. Previously intermittent, the pain had become constant and intense the last three weeks. The major area of unbearable pain complaint was the left lower abdominal area. The pain made sleep impossible. Unable to cope with physical infirmities, he was engulfed with a pall of depression and anxiety.

More than one year earlier, a consultation with another neurologist had revealed the presence of

Parkinson's disease typical symptoms of rigidity and tremor. At that time, the patient overheard the consulting neurologist as he discussed the case with a student in the office. The patient and his wife felt humiliated when the description of "typical deterioration of appearance" was pronounced as though they were not present.

At our initial consultation, depression and anxiety were reported as even greater infirmities than the unbearable abdominal pain. My observation and examination revealed not only signs of Parkinson tremor and rigidity, but a memory deficit greater than expected in a depression or uncomplicated tremor disorder. It was evident that a neurodegenerative process in the brain was clinically presenting early dementia.

Physical examination revealed not only signs of neurodegeneration but also of very elevated systolic blood pressures. Sitting systolic pressures were 50 points higher than desired—in the 170s. Standing systolic blood pressures rose to the 180s. We discussed that depression and anxieties elevated blood pressures, and pain usually elevated blood pressures.

We began a regimen of a starting dose of a second-generation antidepressant with the concomitant administration of a vitamin (L-methylfolate) that would augment and hasten its effectiveness. Also, the L-methylfolate would improve the effectiveness of a previously prescribed anti-Parkinson's tremor medication.

To alleviate the severe back and abdominal pain, laser biostimulation treatment (laser acupuncture) was performed. That treatment utilized optical frequencies that had pain-relieving, tissue-healing, and muscle-relaxation effects. These were applied to appropriate areas on the skin.

The patient departed demonstrating mild clinical improvement. A second session of laser biostimulation was performed two days later. At the conclusion of that treatment, the patient observed that the pain had decreased about 30 percent from a scale of 10/10 to 7/10.

The next day a joint consultation was held with both the patient and his spouse. The previous day's treatment had revealed abdominal pain that was referred from the back and appeared to be intensified by poor posture. It appeared necessary to enlist the wife's assistance in the establishment of an exercise program to improve posture and diminish back pain and spasm. Neither the patient or spouse would accept the concept of a referral to physical therapy. The wife requested oversight, but she rapidly made it known that she did not want her husband's exercise to interfere with her schedule.

A continuation of the laser biostimulation was discussed. The patient stated that his pain was still 7/10, thereby showing a 30 percent reduction after two treatments.

My clinical impression that a newly prescribed antidepressant (desvenlafaxine) was becoming effective was corroborated with improved vital sign readings. (One example was that the systolic blood pressures had dropped from the 180s to the 140s.)

My prognosis was highly optimistic. It appeared that with further laser treatments, within the next two weeks the pain problem would be reasonably well controlled, the depression would be trending to remission, and concurrently a medication regimen for the Parkinson's disease and related neurocognitive degeneration could be integrated.

It was joyful to contemplate a recovery that would restore the patient back to productive activity. Treatments for the back and for the brain demonstrated efficacy in a relatively short span. Necessary exercise routines were not excessive. What a wonderful prognosis!

Two days later, my office received a phone call canceling the next day's appointment. The message left informed me that the patient was discouraged because he was not fully recovered. Further treatment was rejected. I have no information about it ever being obtained from other physicians.

## Carry-Away Lifesavers

Whatever the complexity of your ailments, there may be available remedies.

Realism is necessary in assessing expectations of recovery. Recovery from chronic illnesses is not done with a stopwatch.

Jumping off a ship that is pulling into port does not lead to happy landings.

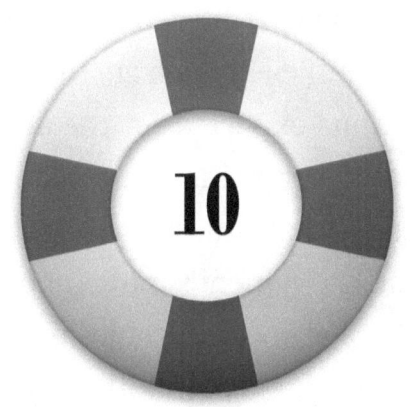

# 10 Lost and Found

A married mother of four children was brought for consultation by her husband. His wife had displayed symptoms of paralyzing depression and had frightening episodes of agitation. Their four children were suffering along with their emotionally disabled mother. There were two children from the patient's previous marriage and two from the current marriage.

This was the second marriage for both husband and wife. In previous years, the patient had succumbed to the advances of an exciting divorced man who convinced her to liberate herself from a "stuffy" husband in exchange for an exciting one. It required years of brain biochemical normalization and psychotherapy sessions before the nature and extent of the exciting new marriage was revealed.

The psychological testing that we performed revealed a severe bipolar depression of sufficient intensity to impair rational conceptualizations expected for the underlying intellectual abilities. The testing results confirmed the clinical impression that mood-stabilizing medications were indicated. The patient's intolerance to lithium carbonate quickly led to acceptable treatment control with carbamapezine (Tegretol). Later relapse responded to the addition of another antidepressant mood stabilizer, Depakote (valproic acid).

The woman's gradual recovery enabled functional restoration. Her responsibilities were resumed; her relationships were reestablished and strengthened; and her marriage and parenting were restored. Happier times returned.

However, it was never all smooth seas and cloudless skies. Though most times were described as being "terribly precious," others were punctuated with emotionally abusive episodes. Periods of intense expression of love were often culminated with revelations of husbandly infidelity. Emotional separations erupted, and reunions reoccurred. No matter how great her wifely devotion and performance, it was never sufficient.

More than a decade later, my patient had not only overcome severe bipolar depression, but she had also conquered previous claustrophobia. For many years she was too fearful to fly in an airplane. She not only overcame that, but she also was able to become a scuba diver. It was almost impossible to believe that she eventually became qualified to teach underwater cave diving—an activity too challenging for many certified scuba divers!

Regardless of my patient's accomplishments, her husband had an unrelenting desire for extramarital relationships. With sons in college, he unilaterally pursued a bachelor's accommodations and lifestyle. The wife's frantic attempts at reconciliation were met with repeated demands for separate lives and separate lovers. That lifestyle was unacceptable to my patient because it conflicted with her concept of parental guidance.

After a second divorce, it was indeed challenging for this woman to regain self-respect and establish an independent lifestyle. Her focus on parenting and her mastery over fearful emotions sustained the post-divorce readjustments. However, it remained too painful to endure frequent encounters with her ex-husband and his paramours. She relocated to a distant state where she had local access to other family members, and this provided comfort and an opportunity to rediscover relationships with fidelity.

## Carry-Away Lifesavers

With commitment to medical care, the most serious emotional difficulties may be controlled and overcome.

Emotional growth and maturation can illuminate where there was darkness.

Not all marriages are made in heaven and are salvageable. Sometimes, marriage failure allows for later voyages to sunnier shores.

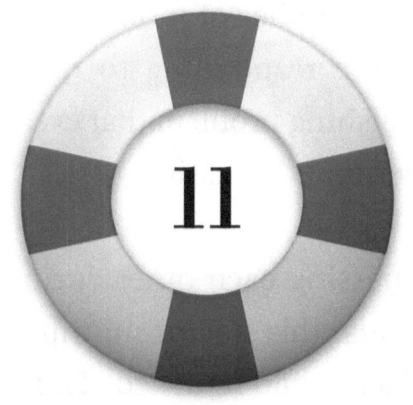

11     Shooting Star

A valued colleague who practiced a subspecialty of internal medicine coordinated with me in the treatment of many patients. He and I assisted each other in rendering care to patients with very complicated illnesses. We enjoyed enormous mutual respect. Over time, we became good friends and our wives demonstrated their culinary excellence to each other.

One morning when our paths crossed during the course of our respective hospital inpatient rounds, he revealed to me that he was suffering from unbearable migraine headaches. He did not want my comprehensive professional care, but he did request that I assist in his mastering the auto-acupressure pain-relieving techniques that he had read in my book (*Quick Headache Relief without Drugs*).

HOWARD D. KURLAND, MD, DLFAPA

After that, he reported for a number of months that the migraine headaches were responding to treatment. They became a diminishing problem that eventually faded away from meriting discussion.

Several years later, while passing each other during the course of hospital rounds, this doctor informed me that his disabling headaches had returned. Those new headaches were not being relieved by the auto-acupressure techniques. Two weeks later, he stated similar complaints.

Each time I heard those complaints, I responded with alarm and offered my professional services. However, these offers were dismissed, along with my other suggestions for diagnostic procedures. When I attempted to discuss his headache issues at other times, my concerns were politely dismissed.

It was only in retrospect that I could appreciate the enormity of the problem. With a patrician background, my colleague was raised with a sense of pride and self-sufficiency. He was an outstanding physician specialist and a leader among his peers. He was chosen to manage a newly conceived large physician practice group. Even among a dozen of his closest friends, no one was aware of his morbid illness.

Apparently, the symptoms of this doctor's headaches were not the same as the previous migraines, but they were related to a devastating illness. His family was at home when a pistol shot was heard resounding from his upstairs bedroom. The head wound was instantly fatal. His funeral was attended by the entire, grieving hospital staff.

There was pervasive depression, and innumerable discussions took place about how we had all failed to help him. I felt (and still feel) that I had failed him. But I am equally certain that the same feelings I was experiencing had to be magnified in his wife, children, and closest friends. I discussed the tragedy with his two closest friends, who were medical colleagues and who both had grown up together with the deceased. Both of these lifelong best friends of the departed professed total unawareness of disease or distress that might have contributed to such a calamitous demise.

My speculation remains that the dramatic finale that culminated in death by suicide was probably related to a fast-growing brain tumor such as a malignant glioblastoma multiforme. There were no symptoms suggestive of the slow-growing "benign" meningiomas that purportedly took the life of the extraordinary musician George Gershwin.

To the best of my knowledge, my friend did not relate the debilitating psychiatric illness that Gershwin had apparently revealed over time on a psychoanalyst's couch. In fact, my departed colleague had not displayed the depressed demeanor, the weight loss, or the concentration difficulties that are typical hallmarks of depressive disease. However, that is just speculation because there was no postmortem examination, and there were no pertinent medical findings to contribute understanding to death by self-inflicted gunshot to the head.

The fact remains that we all witnessed a shooting star—a bright, impressive luminosity that grew rapidly impressive, and just as suddenly, disappeared from our view and into our memories.

# Carry-Away Lifesavers

The difficulties of living with an illness are less than those of the loss of a loved family member.

In dying, as in living, there are meaningful choices and diverse legacies.

The most spectacular performance may be tarnished with a bad finale.

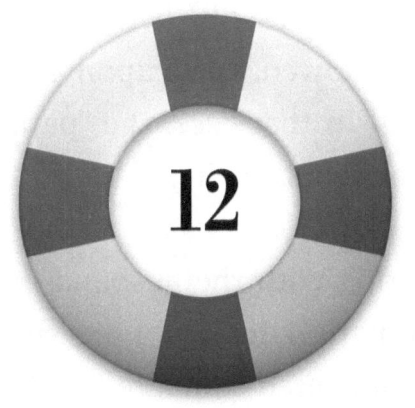

# 12     Change of Course

A middle-aged mother of two early adolescent children sought help with her concerns over an impending divorce. She clearly detailed how her husband had become distant and cold, and how she was absolutely certain that he must be having an affair and would soon request a divorce. Her arguments were convincing. She had been referred to me by her internist, who believed her story and recommended consultation with me.

Earlier in my medical career, I established the need for family corroboration. Years before, a woman presented with what was classic paranoid ideation of that time: being spied on by the Russians, being followed by the Russians, having the Russians tap phone conversations. When I interviewed her husband, he revealed that he was employed on a top-secret government project. The FBI had alerted them that they were being followed, spied upon, and having their phone tapped. In that case, the "paranoid ideation" was not illness but reality.

When I had my first meeting with the husband involved in the then current marital distress, I was surprised at how different he appeared compared to the image that had been described to me. The husband was friendly, talkative, and very concerned about his spouse. He related that she had recently had a total hysterectomy to correct a problem of bleeding from uterine fibroid tumors. Following the surgery, she began to distance herself emotionally. She escalated accusations of marital infidelity. His previously happy household was besieged with *inaccurate accusations of infidelity.*

The husband's appearance was tall, fit, and debonair. It was not surprising that following a hysterectomy, his wife might feel no longer worthy of his attentions because of her perceived lack of sexual desirability.

The husband's expression of true love and absolute commitment to saving his marriage were emphatic. With that support, we held a joint session. The patient was presented with the conflicting evidence, and agreement was reached that she would verify her mental health by undergoing psychological testing.

The projective test results clearly revealed the presence of a significant break with reality, and it confirmed the diagnosis of thought disorder. There was also underlying depression of enormous magnitude. The clinical diagnosis was a classic case of involutional (menopausal) depression with paranoid ideation. In simpler terms, it fit in the spectrum of major depression occurring in the time of sexual hormonal imbalance, which engenders brain neurotransmitter imbalance.

It took several more consultations to convince this distressed wife to accept the concept of illness and treatment. The treatment had to consist of a combination of major tranquilizers (with antipsychotic efficacy) and major antidepressant medications. When the patient finally accepted treatment, she began taking doses of medication. Favorable early response to the medication permitted relatively swift increases to therapeutic levels. Her compliance was excellent, and this enabled me to perform the necessary office monitoring of vital signs and neurological status.

HOWARD D. KURLAND, MD, DLFAPA

The patient's cooperation with psychotherapy was excellent, and her rapid recovery was apparent. Consultations with her husband verified and expedited the recovery. Husband, wife, and children reinstated the previously happy household.

After approximately five years of recovery, the patient expressed concerns about the effect of the economic recession on her husband's business. He had discussed a temporary cash flow problem. Somehow, the patient convinced herself that she had to discontinue quarter yearly consultations with me. She would sacrifice those reevaluations in order to repay her husband's sacrifices during her former time of illness. Also, this patient felt that she could get her medication prescriptions from her internist without the additional cost of psychiatric monitoring.

She asserted that she was fully recovered and capable of sustaining that recovery. I expressed my concerns that the sacrificing might be indicative of the grandiose act of behaving like a martyr; and therefore, such conceptualization might be indicative of relapsing paranoid ideation.

My concerns about relapse potential were expressed first to the patient and then to the husband. Then, I discussed relapse concerns with the internist who had agreed to write the prescriptions for the psychiatric medications. I made a clear request to be notified about symptoms of relapse.

About three years later, I received a telephone call from her husband. His wife had stopped her medication over the previous six months. The internist had issued yearly prescriptions, and he had no way of being aware of the medication discontinuation. Unfortunately, the wife's emotional illness returned.

This time, the husband was caught unprepared. He was served with divorce papers for a divorce that he did not want. He was informed that his wife's matrimonial attorneys were prepared to contest any psychiatric evaluations requested. He expressed his sense of disappointment and defeat, but he felt unable to reverse the impending legal defeat.

Several years later, I learned that her then ex-husband had adapted successfully after the divorce. His children were angry with their mother, but they found solace in the care and custody of their father. In the following year, at the insistence of his children, he began to seek new feminine companionship. Their mother disintegrated into her chosen world of mental illness.

## Carry-Away Lifesavers

When one has the courage to accept help, recovery is usually expedited.

If it is not broken, don't fix it. If your current medical regimen produces optimal results, do not interfere with it.

If your physician recommends reasonable follow-up care, wisdom dictates heeding that advice.

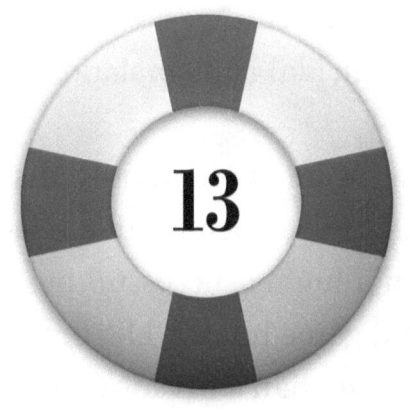

# 13

# Vessel Sunk by Friendly Fire

A forty-year-old man was referred by another patient to obtain relief from unremitting lower back pain. At the time of the initial evaluation, he related that family stress issues seemed to play havoc with his back. He noticed that the emotional stresses were having a very negative effect on his mental and physical health.

Intensifying physical and mental problems were overwhelming. His back pain reportedly interfered with sleep. A prescription of anti-inflammatory corticosteroids by an orthopedic specialist intensified his sleep problems. He began to have problems both falling asleep and staying asleep. Physical pain interfered with his struggling with family issues, and the inability to cope increased his despondency. He had become increasingly claustrophobic, and his interest in any pleasurable activity vanished. Agonizing back spasms led to despair and suicidal contemplation.

These dramatic symptoms were more vividly distressing when viewed from the perspective that relatively recently he had been a highly successful businessman, athlete, pilot, and game hunter. His initial back injury had occurred more than a decade earlier, after slipping and falling on a hard tennis court. Multiple physician consultations had not provided relief from his current intolerable symptoms. His obvious suffering was observed by a tradesman who was working on a home repair. That tradesman related the recovery he had obtained from a doctor in a far-distant suburb. He convincingly argued that the lengthy commute would be worth the effort.

Because of the complexity of the physical emotional problems, we agreed on a comprehensive evaluation. Physical examinations and laboratory evidence such as X-rays and MRIs were correlated. Psychological testing was performed, and the relevant information was integrated with pertinent data obtained from psychotherapy sessions. The clinical picture was that of physical illness intertwined with emotional distress and brain biochemical imbalance. To resolve these problems, the patient would be required to follow a combination of physical treatments, medications, and psychotherapy.

The very distressing family problems were related to a family business. This patient's father had founded a hugely successful insurance agency, and the sons were incorporated as business partners. An irreparable dispute arose between my patient and the other family members–business partners. Illegal business activities were uncovered by my shocked patient, but he could not get other family members to remedy the situation. Unable to tolerate such illegal, immoral behavior, my patient went to court and filed a lawsuit that requested termination of undesirable business practices.

Imagine the distress of someone who felt so principled that he had to file legal redress against the successful corporation that he owned jointly with his father and brothers. During the previous years, they had enjoyed a close, caring family structure. Now the idyllic picture was being erased with uncharacteristic animosity. The successful son who was an athlete, pilot, and wild-game hunter was now enveloped in legal combat with his beloved family of origin.

To treat this man's biochemical depression, I pre-scribed a combination of antidepressant medications. Panic attacks were frequent companions to the emo-tional turmoil swirling around the legal battleground. Both symptoms of depression and panic disorder of-ten respond to treatment with antidepressants, which have a significant effect on serotonin. Fluoxetine (Prozac) was effective in ameliorating the patient's daytime symptoms, and trazodone (Desyrel) assisted him in getting sleep at night.

He received back pain relief with acupuncture-related treatments. Laser biostimulation was the most effec-tive treatment. Activity-related pain exacerbations at home were controlled with a TENS (transcutaneous electrostimulation) unit.

Psychotherapeutic efforts for this man included pains-taking sessions of discovery, analysis, emotional ca-tharsis, perceptive reconstruction, and reformulation. In those sessions, issues were deconstructed and re-constructed into usable perspectives. My patient's life first became tolerable again, and then progressed back to pleasurable.

Starting a new insurance business would be sufficiently challenging, and creating a successful new enterprise in a year would appear to be an impossible goal. However, this man accomplished these seemingly impossible tasks despite the fact that he had residual physical pain limitations and was still challenged by episodic emotional disruptions. His unblemished reputation for fairness and honesty resounded in the business world. This, along with his friendly charisma, accelerated the man's financial success.

When his wife was unable to bear children, he came to terms with the loss of his desired dreams of parenting. Unfortunately, this gave impetus to returning to ever-more-dangerous athletic endeavors. During the next decade, he had a number of injuries that would alter his life.

More than a decade after our initial consultation, a friend of my patient had offered him a lesson in motorcycle riding. The supervision of his initiation to motorcycles was particularly inadequate. My patient sustained a fall, fracturing his ankle and re-creating an unbearably painful back. Surgery was performed on the ankle fracture.

After the course of postoperative recovery and re-habilitation, the patient and his wife went on a fishing vacation. They were enjoying the pleasures of a rented fishing boat in calm Canadian waters when the patient's seat suddenly became loose. He was hurtled through the windshield of the boat and struck his lower back on the hull during the fall. The next day, his vacation had to be terminated because of back pain and disability.

The local orthopedist first attempted to control the back pains with transforaminal epidural steroid injections. Physical therapy and opioid pain medications were added. After months of suffering, an extensive orthopedic surgery was proposed. A spinal fusion surgery was performed, and an extensive bracing system was installed.

The surgery failed to relieve the pain. There were again multiple medical consultations, which finally resulted in management by a local pain clinic. The person of responsibility for prescribing pain medications at the pain clinic was not a physician, but a nurse practitioner. Eventually, the nurse practitioner prescribed a long-acting, strong opiate skin patch named Duragesic (fentanyl).

Dosing with fentanyl patches needs to be done carefully. Doses should be adjusted no more frequently than three days after the initial dose, and every six days thereafter. Patients should be monitored; however, this was not the care rendered. The nurse practitioner escalated the dose with unsafe rapidity.

When the patient's wife called the nurse practitioner in the middle of the night to report with alarm that her husband looked comatose, the nurse's advice was to let him sleep at home through the night. His wife called an ambulance in the morning to transport the comatose husband to the hospital. He never revived. The report of the county coroner documented the details.

This shockingly tragic death was the result of medical care rendered under the supposed supervision of physicians who gave opiate-prescribing responsibility to a nurse practitioner with inadequate training and poor judgment. It is distressing to wonder how often this may occur in the future with the economic push to utilize nonphysicians to provide "economical" medical care.

The loss to society of this valuable man is irreparable. But he left a legacy of brilliance, uncompromising integrity, devoted friendship, and the ability to overcome adversity. The ironic consolation of his tragic demise was to conceptualize it as a protection from further betrayals by people in whom he placed trust.

It is not difficult to recall the biblical allegory ("I will be betrayed three times before the cock crows") of an exceptionally caring, giving, charismatic man receiving a final betrayal before dawn that led to a death sentence. Perhaps that allegory extends to the daily refusals by nonphysician medical payers to provide lifesaving care requested by caring physicians.

## Carry-Away Lifesavers

Trust is an essential component of a happy, productive life. But trust must be carefully awarded and periodically reevaluated.

Hopefully, one is raised with trustworthy parents who teach us that the concept of "trust in the Lord" is different than an absolute, unquestioning trust of the judgment of others.

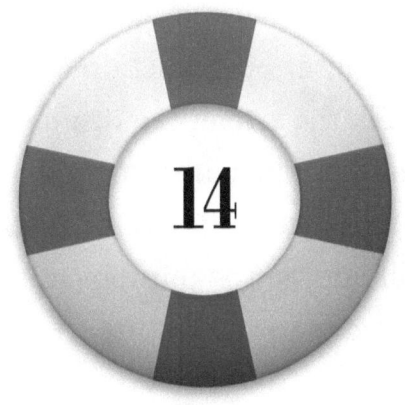

# 14

# In Transit at an Idyllic Port

The internist caring for this mother of five adopted children was adamant about her receiving psychiatric care for alcoholism. Her consumption of alcohol was staggering. She was usually intoxicated. Her husband could not run a professional career and be a stay-at-home parent. The family finances were being consumed in alcoholic excess.

The out-of-the-home, in-the-world presentation made by this patient was impressive. Expensive attire and obvious beautician care was displayed with a pleasant demeanor. The external facade was soon revealed to be the socially acceptable presentation that made the acquisition of alcohol obtainable. This woman was using alcoholic intoxication to anesthetize the torments of unbearable mental illness.

It was quickly apparent that this was a very tortured being. Alcoholism was an engrafted addiction, and this woman had acquired it in the attempt to disguise and to cope with schizophrenia. Most amazing to me was her ability to hide her psychotic demons for so many years. The clinical diagnosis was reinforced by indisputable findings on psychometric testing.

She was able to undergo intense comprehensive diagnosis and treatment protocols because of the strong encouragement of her family. The use of major antipsychotic medications was essential to institute a process of neurotransmitter rebalancing. Alcoholic withdrawal was paramount, and the prevention of seizures and delirium was required. The body's vitamins and minerals that had been depleted because of the alcohol needed to be restored. In addition, her brain and body needed detoxification.

Even more complex was the unraveling of the underlying emotional disorder. We were confronted with solving the problems of family relationships. Her parents were deceased, and the family suburban mansion had been bequeathed to her. It was her husband and five adopted children that now resided with her there.

The children had been adopted because the couple desired a family despite the inability to conceive a child. Overcoming the emotional pain, shame, and guilt that disguised the origin of this problem took almost four years of treatment. The problem was not fertility; it was frigidity. Marital sexuality was blemished with horrors of parental childhood rape. This tortured woman was residing in the home where her father had maternal approval to rape his daughter. The rapes occurred frequently from the time of childhood, and they only desisted when she became engaged to be married.

These recollections of paternal incest were not psychotic ideation. I was able to return them to consciousness only through laborious psychotherapeutic efforts. Slowly the maze of the tortured past became visible and passable. In the course of time, other family members verified the horrifying details. During these family revelations and verifications, I shared the discomfiture of the victim.

Suffering through the psychotherapy, the patient was rewarded with previously unknown health. Her marital sexual life became exciting and rewarding. At long last, she became pregnant. She carried the baby to term and delivered a son. Now there was an ecstatic mother and father.

The joys of parenthood may sometimes be a mixed blessing. Child rearing can become too much on occasion, and the most amiable disposition may be taxed by an overly rambunctious child. Their later-in-life conceived son was never a usual child. By the time of entrance into preschool, he was noted to be unusually selfish and combative. By second grade, he was a regular on the detention lists. He could not be helped by school psychologists. Thus, as a preadolescent, he was brought to my office by his parents.

My impression was that of a young "Dennis the Menace." It was probable that his peers saw him as attractive and perceived his rebelliousness as appealing. He was cooperative in evaluation. Much to my chagrin, both my clinical data and psychometric testing data suggested the absence of a moral conscience and the diagnosis of sociopathy (antisocial personality disorder). Whatever was attempted therapeutically was ineffective. The boy had no motivation or desire to change.

During the middle of his high school years, it was my painful duty to inform the parents that I concluded their son may be an untreatable sociopath. He was already into the use and distribution of drugs. With distressed emotions, I predicted that drug-related activities might end his life before his twenty-first year. I had never before and have never since been required to make such a horrible prediction.

My prediction was unfortunately only slightly incorrect. According to the coroner's report, six months after his twenty-first birthday, his life was ended by a murderer's gunshot to the chest during a drug-related dispute.

Working through the loss of an only naturally born son would be difficult enough for a mother with no history of schizophrenia and alcoholism. In this case, some of this woman's illness episodes recurred and were treated. But there was no deterioration to previous illness levels. However, the enormity of the emotional trauma may have been a contributing factor to the development of an autoimmune disorder. Two years later, she perished from heart disease. Before her demise, she had rescued years of happiness from the pits of despair.

The family love and devotion that supported the recovery of a chronic schizophrenic alcoholic was wonderful to observe. Painful revelations had enabled this woman to recover. The replication of the sociopathic father in the sociopathic grandson was enormously gruesome. However, my patient's years of recovery and the evolution of reasonable harmony in her marriage were blissful to behold.

## Carry-Away Lifesavers

Overcoming some of life's problems may require an enormous amount of "true grit," but greater efforts bring more glorious victories.

When we support the recovery of our loved ones, we are giving a gift that also enriches ourselves and our future.

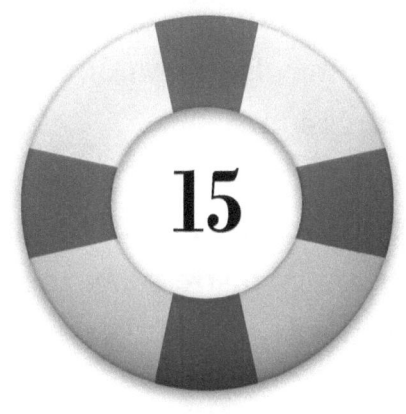

# 15

# Twenty-One-Gun Salute

A married mother of five children was experiencing difficult times. She had experienced the removal of two breast tumors fifteen years earlier. Now she was in her midfifties.

Her complaints of anxiety and depression were so significant that her internist had insisted on consultation with a neuropsychiatrist. There was a history of serious depressive disease in both her father and brother. The father had recovered only after a course of ECT (electroconvulsive therapy).

Significant current family stressors were active. One son was divorcing and remarrying. Another was waging a feud with his father and refusing to speak with either parent. Her husband had developed hypertension, and her menopause was symptomatic.

Psychological testing identified multiple emotional issues requiring attention. Testing also was indicative of underlying biological depression.

Frequent recall of dreams was especially useful in elucidating the nature of emotional distress. We then devised and adopted problem-solving strategies.

But the underlying biological anxiety-depressive mood issues were much more troubling. It was difficult to imagine that whatever type of antidepressant and/or mood stabilizer and/or major tranquilizer and/or minor tranquilizer was prescribed, undesirable side effects necessitated discontinuation.

Klonopin (clonazepam) is an anticonvulsant benzo-diazepine. Although scientifically considered a minor (rather than major) tranquilizer, it alone provided major relief of anxiety and reasonable diminution of depressive symptomatology. Moreover, it continued to provide moderate efficacious effects without undesired side effects for more than twenty years.

What tragedy might befall a mother graver than the loss of her firstborn and "perfect" son? Cancer struck and relentless metastatic progression caused unspeakable agony. After a series of medical heroics, the unthinkable occurred. A son full of sociability, good humor, and artistic talents was now a painfully blessed memory.

Within the following year, the older of her two daughters noticed a mole enlarging on her thigh. A melanoma was diagnosed. Metastatic progression developed rapidly. The daughter was unresponsive to treatment, and the metastatic melanoma led to a rapid termination of life.

Now two of the five children were around only in memory and dreams. Both parents were in emotional shock. The remaining three children were also afflicted with emotional distress. Surviving the death of two siblings to cancer and having parents who lost two children to cancer was unbearable.

Religious conviction, outstanding pastoral support, and a wonderfully comforting church congregation helped sustain her ability to continue her roles as wife, mother, and grandmother. She also continued twice-weekly consultation enabling our identification and confrontation of troubled emotions.

A most outstanding behavior was her perpetual endeavor to be warm and giving to others. She be-
friended others of all ages. One younger female
church congregant developed an especially close
mother-daughter-like relationship. The three children of this young friend wanted to be regarded a
"grandchildren" and expressed their sentiments with
invitations to "grandmother visiting days" at school.

As the next decade passed, the acute pain of the
grieving subsided in the emotions. However, a back
disorder led to a spinal nerve root compression,
which the patient experienced as pain in the side of
the abdominal wall. Relief was obtained by twice
weekly sessions of spinal manipulation. Those visits
to the chiropractor's office enabled a warm personal
friendship with a caregiver who was about the age of
her deceased son. Thereby, relationships were continued with her three surviving children and also
with replacement surrogates for the deceased son
and daughter.

Grocery clerks, doctors' staffs, and household em-
ployees were always treated with the highest regard,
and they responded in the same fashion. She was
generous with verbal praise, with economic gifts to

those in need, and to those whom she felt should have life made a little easier financially. Her generosity was such that family members became concerned about the amount.

A few years shy of two decades after the demise of her two children, and early in the ninth decade of life, a disturbance in cardiac rhythm began intermittent interruptions in adequate blood flow to the brain. She received cardiological consultation, but no successful treatment availed.

Two more tragedies were unfolding: her beloved husband was besieged by cancer, and her "special" daughter-in-law was perishing from cancer-related illness.

Despite all her life's difficulties, lying in a hospital bed, she expressed gratitude for all the joys that life had afforded her. Her cardiac conduction problems (broken heart) resulted in her demise. I am sure that she passed away "counting her blessings."

# Carry-Away Lifesavers

An awareness of family medical problems allows "an ounce of prevention rather than a pound of cure."

When your hurts seem overwhelming, try to obtain perspective that others have survived their personal holocaust.

Sometimes your body will reject the medication that works for almost everybody else. Let your physician assist in discovering what may be the innovative solution for you.

Emotional generosity is rewarding to the giver and is more often rewarded in kind.

Appreciating what you have (rather than what you do not have) is the basis of a happy life.

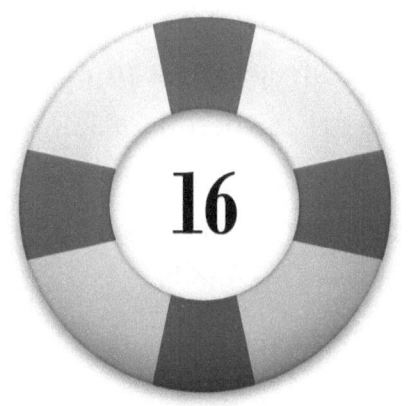

## 16      Attention on Deck

Now hear this: the CDC (Centers for Disease Control) estimates that 25 percent of all adult males and 10 percent of all adult females have brain oxygen deprivation syndromes related to obstruction of the airways during sleep (obstructive sleep apnea). It is commonly experienced by the sleeping partner's hearing loud snoring, which is followed by a cessation of breathing sounds, which is then followed by a silent interval that is punctuated by a loud snort.

There are other causes of sleep apnea such as central sleep apnea, which is caused by a brain control dysfunction.

Adverse effects related to sleep apnea include excessive daytime sleepiness, decreased work productivity, and significantly increased risk of heart attack and stroke. Moreover, current estimates state that there is a 25 percent probability of sleep apnea in adults desiring elective surgery and that there is a failure to diagnose sleep apnea in 80 percent of patients at the time of surgery. It is thought that sleep apnea increases the risk of complications during surgery and during the post-surgical recovery period.

Sleep apnea also has been found in children of all ages. The actual incidence percentage is not currently known. (One does not see what one does not look for.)

Usually the treatment of sleep apnea is relatively uncomplicated and inexpensive. Obstructive sleep apnea can often be controlled with an inexpensive, nonprescription dental appliance or inexpensive chinstrap. Even when CPAP (continuous positive air pressure) or related devices are necessary during sleep, it may involve only a small bedside unit and cloth nasal mask. The risk of complications is high for all who refuse to recognize the necessity to treat sleep apnea.

Absolute, adamant refusal to treat sleep apnea was the situation of a sixty-five-year-old male who recently perished with a massive coronary during sleep. Also, a forty-five-year-old female, who was not hypertensive, had a stroke.

## Carry-Away Lifesavers

Ignoring the exceptionally common disorder of sleep apnea is enormously perilous.

Treatment of obstructive sleep apnea is usually very inexpensive. It is always much less expensive than a funeral (or even life as an invalid).

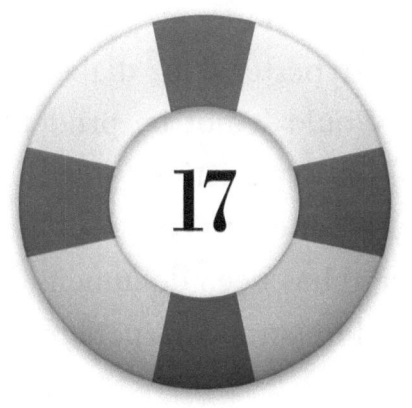

# 17 Disembarkation

Senior crew going ashore need to be aware that neurodegeneration (pathological aging processes in the brain) occurs in almost everyone after forty-five years of age. What is politely called "growing old" may be growing ill. The decline in memory function, analysis, and problem solving may be related to an ill brain, not just an aging brain.

The 2013 edition of Diagnostic Manual prepared by the American Psychiatric Association contains a newly minted diagnosis label of "mild neurocognitive disorder." This refers to early clinical manifestations of impairment that often precede the development of major neurocognitive disorders such as the senile dementias.

Preventative treatments are commonly accepted for medical disorders such as hypertension, diabetes, and elevated cholesterol. Would it not be prudent to apply prevention for brain dysfunction? For the last several decades in my practice, the appropriate application of early treatment has been documented to be impressively successful in compliant patients.

Help is already here. First in order is the medical control of physical ailments that are potentially enormously brain-damaging. An undernourished body has an undernourished brain. The brain needs both adequate nourishment and adequate exercise. Abnormally elevated blood sugar levels significantly increase the risk of dementia in both diabetic and non-diabetic seniors.

Blood pressure must be reasonably controlled so that it is not hypertensive (too high) or hypotensive (too low) in either sitting or standing positions.

Blood oxygen levels must be adequate. These are easily measured quickly from a small device placed over the finger called an oximeter. Lung disease, sleep apnea, blocked arteries, or blood clots may deprive the brain of adequate oxygen.

It is important to control heart rhythm abnormalities, and the need for an anticoagulant should be assessed to prevent clots being thrown to the brain. Arteries in the heart and brain need to be open and functioning; elevated blood fat levels of bad cholesterol and high triglycerides require identification and treatment. Anemias are obviously dangerous to the brain.

At the senior age level, deficient vitamin B12 levels may lead to irreversible nervous system damage. Thyroid abnormalities must be corrected before irreversible brain damage occurs. Deficient vitamin D levels require correction, but these are usually not as devastating to the brain as deficiencies of vitamin B12 or thyroid hormone.

Increased fluid levels inside the brain may cause compression death of brain cells. This disorder is called internal hydrocephalus. Diagnosis of the disorder is indicated by a history of symptoms and is often identifiable on a brief, basic neurological exam. If considered, diagnostic brain studies such as MRIs may be both brain-saving and lifesaving.

Untreated psychiatric depression is related to diminished levels of BDNF (brain derived neurotrophic factor) with subsequent loss of structure and function. Antidepressant medications variably increase BDNF levels and are associated with brain tissue restoration.

Other neurodegenerative disorders such as Parkinson's disease and Lou Gehrig's disease (ALS: amyotrophic lateral sclerosis) require not only their specific treatments but also consideration of treatment for neurocognitive issues.

When the underlying medical disorders have been identified and medical corrections commenced, the following treatment protocols may provide dramatic results:

Initiate (or continue) daily doses of 15 mg of the oral vitamin L-methylfolate. This active metabolite of folic acid is essential for brain health, but it cannot be obtained from taking plain folic acid (a toxic dose of folic acid would be required).

A NMDA (N-methyl-D-aspartate) receptor antagonist such as memantadine is generally added next and titrated to maintenance doses.

Subsequently, a central acetylcholinesterase inhibitor such as donepezil, galantine, or rivastigmine is added as a third agent and titrated to maintenance doses.

The above order has proven highly effective. Reversing the order and adding memantadine last is ordinarily not efficacious. Foundations need to be laid before upper floors are improved.

After the foundation treatment is established, other prescription medical foods that improve cerebral glucose metabolism such as caprylidine have demonstrated added efficacy.

## Carry-Away Lifesavers

It is not a kindness to yourself to deny brain degeneration and mislabel it as aging. Normally, the brain begins neurodegeneration after age forty-five.

Even if you have little evident impairment, do you wish to discover how long you can go without severe impairment?

Your parents undoubtedly introduced the ancient wisdom of a "healthy mind in a healthy body."

A few simple remedies taken in a timely fashion may enable "being there" for children, grandchildren, and maybe even great-grandchildren.

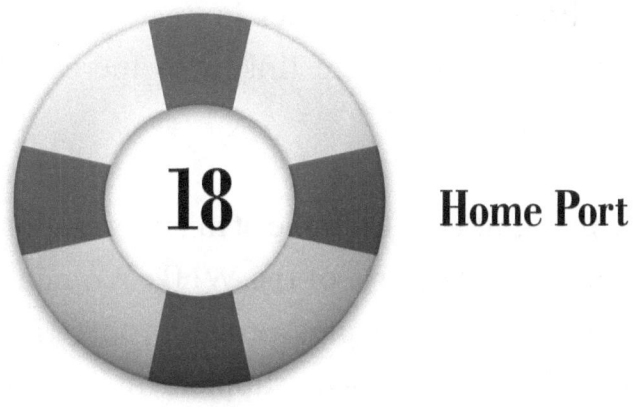

**18**  Home Port

A board ship, food is prepared in the galley. At home, it is important that you do not become a galley slave. Nutritional intake that is sensible served man well over the centuries. Fad diets and government advice are always questionable and usually subject to substantial change.

Former government nutritional advice contributed to an overconsumption of white pastas, which has been linked to epidemic obesity. Nutritional experts panicked the public away from butter to substitute margarines, which were legislated against five decades later when it was discovered the substitutes had potentially deadly trans fats.

Trans fats are polyunsaturated fats that can raise levels of LDL (bad cholesterol), and lower levels of

HDL (good cholesterol). Increases in heart attacks, strokes, and death rates were linked to increased intake of trans fats.

Another highly significant example of misinformation was the 2002 faulty analysis of the WHI (Women's Health Initiative) estrogen plus progesterone trial. The beneficial effect of estrogen supplementation in reducing mortality after hysterectomy was initially overlooked. Current 2013 studies have concluded that over the past decade, thousands of postmeno-pausal women had premature deaths related to the lack of estrogen therapy after hysterectomy.

The difference between a medicine and a poison is dose. The same drug (Coumadin: generic is war-farin) is sold as a rat poison and as a therapeutic anticoagulant.

For most people without a specific sensitivity or in-tolerance, one alcoholic drink daily consumed with food is both brain and heart healthy.

According to physical status, there is a minimum number of food calories and salt intake necessary for good health. Because of faulty information, salt restriction has led to problems with hyponatremia (low blood sodium levels) sometimes contributing to hypotension (low blood pressure) symptoms of light-headedness, dizziness, fainting, and tissue injury.

Fish oil supplements have been promoted as heart healthy for their omega-3 content. However, large daily doses (greater than 1000–2000 mg) have been associated with significantly increased incidence of prostate cancer. Of course, if the fish oils are not certified to be free from mercury contamination, that poses a possible neurotoxic hazard.

Inspection of "private areas" for skin cancers may save your life. An estimated 20% of Americans will develop skin cancers such as melanomas. Melanomas can occur in genital areas, under fingernails, under toenails, and on the soles of the feet. Inspection should be done on skin areas where the sun shines and also where it does not shine. Look for a skin growth that has increased in size and appears black, brown, multicolored or translucent. It is wise to con-sult a dermatologist if a mole or any brown spot changes color, texture, shape, and/or size.

Bunk time is essential, but it is not exercise. Although the recommended healthy expression of sensual pleasures in bunk-related activities is favorable for health maintenance, it does not produce fitness on deck. Prolonged sitting in front of a television or computer screen for uninterrupted hours can be deadly.

A short (10 to 20 minutes) afternoon nap, especially before 4 p.m., can be refreshing. Nap times of 30 to 60 minutes may cause unpleasant groggy feelings after awakening. A slightly upright sleeping position for naps helps to avoid deep sleep. If one has sleep apnea it is prudent to skip afternoon naps.

Walking is recommended as healthy exercise. Post-surgical patients are instructed to walk so that peristalsis (intestinal movement) gets restored. Bones require weight-bearing to maintain their strength; demineralization occurs with lack of weight-bearing. Studies have shown that fifty minutes of brisk walking five days per week is usually the best rehabilitation for peripheral artery disease.

Walking is much less stressful on the body than running. The use of two walking sticks mobilizes shoulders, arms, and wrist activity, and may contribute an additional 30 percent more caloric expenditure to the walking effort. Walking on the ground is regarded as producing more positive health rewards than using a treadmill.

For chair-bound individuals, there are apps for your smart phone that will give complete exercise routines while seated. There is a multiplicity of free apps for seven-minute exercise routines.

The use of a personal electronic device to monitor activity may be quite helpful in recording actual physical energy expended. Such small, convenient devices are frequently marketed as fitness recorders. They are relatively inexpensive.

At home, health monitoring is usually relatively simple and often more important than testing done elsewhere. Blood sugars can be obtained relatively rapidly and painlessly at home. The cost of testing is much less than in commercial labs. Blood pressures accurately monitored at home have been demonstrated to be more meaningful and useful than those obtained outside the home environment.

Using electronic sensors to monitor the safety of our dwellings is a well established practice. Home perimeters can be guarded electronically. Heat levels, carbon dioxide levels, and competency of electrical systems can be continuously monitored. Now that technology has extended to monitor the occupants, it is surprising to hear patients decline the use of home health monitors often, even after arriving for their visits with the assistance of such devices in their automobiles.

The smartphone is more than an iPhone or android device; it is potentially a mobile medical office. Easily available and relatively inexpensive attachments are available to monitor blood pressure, heart rate, heart rhythm, and electrocardiograms. Simple attachments can monitor breathing and blood pressure, thereby enabling the assessment of emotional states and facilitating personal control. A personal wearable sensor for the back can be purchased and paired with a free iPhone app to monitor improper posture. One can utilize the smartphone as a "doc in the pocket."

It would be remiss to leave home port without the usual trite admonition that the enjoyment of comforts at home should include an awareness of the potential of the dangers at home. A relaxed attitude at the top of a ladder may lead to an unwanted consequence.

Cooking with gas is gourmet; burning yourself is not. Attempting to work with electric wiring without proper knowledge of color coding can be explosive. A hair dryer falling into water may be electrifying or deadly. Rational thought and behavior belong on both sides of your doorways.

"Time is brain" is a current (2013) operational concept in neurology. The expression "time is brain" is meant to convey the urgency to administer blood clot–dissolving agents such as TPA in a timely fashion. Using agents to improve blood flow within the first two hours after a stroke is thought to be optimal window of time. A similar concept applies after an acute heart attack, when it might be said that "time is heart."

It can be critical to use emergency service transport. Identification of symptoms of stroke and/or heart attack is often time-critical. Here again, the utilization of information from your smartphone, tablet, or computer may be lifesaving.

There are numerous apps to assist. Free apps that give information on triage can be easily accessed. Although a useful free app such as iTriage may be downloaded at any time, it is strongly recommended to preload such apps in preparation for a possible emergency while in home port or away.

Symptoms such as the acute loss of equilibrium with the tendency to lurch to one side may be indicative of stroke, especially with the compromise of the posterior brain circulation in such main blood vessels as the vertebral arteries. A triage app affords easy and rapid assistance in evaluating symptoms that may require a 911 call for emergency skilled medical attention.

## Carry-Away Lifesavers

Home is where the health is.

Awareness of risky behaviors may be lifesaving both at home and away.

You can live better with electronics, especially with an awareness of medical apps.

Cast off anchors of denial. By gaining weighty medical information and revisiting life perspective, your voyage may be longer, allowing you to reach more desirable shores.

www.ingramcontent.com/pod-product-compliance
Lightning Source LLC
Chambersburg PA
CBHW030813180526
45163CB00003B/1270